# Believe 271....A Story About Cancer in the Fire Service

## Changing the Culture

### Chief Brian McQueen

Published by FastPencil

Published by FastPencil
307 Orchard City Drive
Suite 210
Campbell CA 95008 USA
info@fastpencil.com
(408) 540-7571
(408) 540-7572 (Fax)
http://www.fastpencil.com

This book represents information obtained throughout this firefighter's battle with occupational cancer. They reflect the beliefs of he and his family.

Printed in the United States of America.

First Edition

*Dedicating of this book goes to so many. To my wife Sarah, my rock that walked with me each step of my cancer treatments. I would not be able to write this book if it wasn't for her love. To my son Ryan, his wife Erin, my brother Bob and his wife Nancy, my nephew Lieutenant Joseph McQueen, the Flisnik family, thank you for giving me the love needed to make the trek each week to NYC for treatments and for the prayers said daily for my recovery. Thank you Sister Dolorosa Lenk, my aunt who proofed this book for me. Special thanks to Dan and Betsy Schwertfeger who pushed me to get treatment away from home. The daily cards Betsy gave me to open after each treatment would bring tears to my eyes. They were absolutely correct. To my fire service brotherhood you all are special to me. My Whitesboro CSD family, there is no better a group then you. Carla Ryan and Wendy Karas, your weekly cards and daily prayers were so well needed. Finally, to the Believe 271 Foundation and their loved ones, we are doing great things for those less fortunate.*

❧

# Acknowledgments

Thanks to my physician Dr. Toby Taylor and his staff, these people are second to none. To the medical staff and oncology department at Memorial Sloan Kettering Cancer Center, thank you. To the brotherhood of the fire service in Oneida, Herkimer and New York State, thank you for walking this fight with me. Finally, to the Believe 271 Foundation Inc., you had a dream to help others, you have grown this dream to be one of the most respective foundations for firefighters across this great nation. You Gotta Believe!

# CONTENTS

# 1

## THE BACKGROUND BEHIND THE VOLUNTEER

Growing up in a small village in central New York named Yorkville, with
two older brothers, I grew fond of
my neighbor down the street named
Mark Waterman. Mark's sons were
great friends of mine, we played
street ball together on Highland
Ave., went to Sacred Heart Elementary school together, and spent many
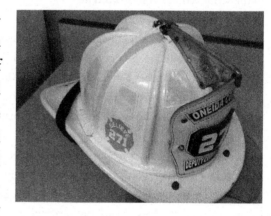
nights doing sleepovers at each other's homes.
What truly amazed me though with the Waterman family was the unending
dedication the father, Mark Waterman, had for the Yorkville
Volunteer Fire Department. No matter whatever time of day and night the.
Bell hit for an alarm, Mark left what he was doing around the house and
assisted a community resident in need of help. You see, Mark was a pioneer in
the EMS field in Oneida County, so the officers and members of YFD needed
his knowledge for at that time the calls were named, Inhalator Calls.

Mark would return home and share some of his experience, that which he could without
giving away private information, and it was those stories that lit the fire during the year of
1973, at a young age of 18, to begin to think about becoming a volunteers firefighter. After
graduating from Notre Dame High School, my inspirations carried me through the summer
months preparing daily for my college career.

That August I packed my bags for college, Daemen College in Amherst, NY, to begin my post secondary education in hopes of fulfilling my dream to become an elementary teacher and coach. This small non-Sectarian school in Western New York offered me my time to grow and actually pave a path for my future.

I met some wonderful way friends there, Michael Arcuri, Randy Gerlach, Luis Santiago , Anthony DeMatteo, just to name a few. I joined the Phi Beta Gamma fraternity on campus and worked in the college's Rathskeller as a bartender. My Senior year I was a Resident Assistant for primarily our "fraternity dorm." While in college I had an opportunity to manage the student athletic department scheduling, played two years of basketball and four years of flag football. My body has never really recovered from that flag football league! Throughout my student teaching experiences I met some great sport figures like members of the French Connection for the Buffalo Sabres, as well as Marv Levy, all who had children or relatives in some of the schools that I volunteered in.

Even though I was away from Yorkville, I still had that urge to become a " Mark Waterman." That volunteer firefighter who answered the cries for help no matter the time of day or weather outside. So one day I drove my Plymouth Duster, oh what a beast that car was, to the Snyder Volunteer Fire Department on Main Street in Amherst, NY, to talk with them about the volunteer fire service. From that day forward, their doors were always open to me and I spent countless hours assisting them at various events, washing trucks and just watching TV.

In April of 1977, my hero, my father suffered his third heart attack. I will never forget the call from my brother Tom, you need to go home, "it's not good." I made home just in time to say good bye to my dad at St. Luke's Hospital. See my dad was an avid smoker and took his job very seriously, thus providing him with a lot of stress. My mom was devastated, and I knew that she would want me home after graduation.

Following my graduation from Daemen, I returned home to search for an elementary education job. I spoke with Mark Waterman and asked him if it would be worth my while to join the Yorkville FD or wait to see where my employment takes me. The latter was his suggestion. With no jobs in the area, I interviewed at York Central School in Retsof, NY and was offered a third grade position and the Assistant a Junior Varsity Football position. I accepted the position, much to the dismay of my mother, but I needed to get my foot in the door as education was changing.

I loved that job! I worked with two wonderful ladies at the grade level, and one of them owned and operated the Truck Stop and Cafe next to the school with her husband, so meals were of a premium. They treated me like her son.

As for the coaching, my first year opened my eyes to one of the powerhouse schools in NYS football, Caledonia- Mumford, the Mount Union of high school football. I truly enjoyed the coaching staff and the students and looked forward to our Thursday afternoon JV games and Friday Night football in Retsof.

While at York Central I lived in a one room apartment behind a garage in Leicester, N.Y. The lady that owned it was named "Jenks" had a ton of children and was an outstanding baker. The Leicester FD was only a half a mile from the apartment, so in my free time, I would spend some time at their station, assisting them with fundraisers, washing trucks and helping them when they returned from a call. As you can tell, I still had that Mark Waterman urge to help others.

Throughout my year at York, my mother was passionate for me to return home and be with her. The loss of my dad was not settling to well with her. So in the spring I applied to the Oriskany Central School District for a third grade position, interviewed in front of a great educational leader in Norma Harter and then with Superintendent Ken Gadbow. One week following my interview, Mrs. Harter called me in York and informed me that the position was mine. In fact, I would be taking the place of one of Sarah's friends, Roberta Farr, who reminds Sarah every time she sees her that it was because of her move out of Oriskany is the reason we met.

I was finally coming home! Mr. Bernie Block, the Athletic Director at Oriskany contacted me and asked me to be his Assistant Varsity Football Coach as well. God was truly looking over me.

I met some of the greatest, students, parents, teachers and community members from Oriskany. This opportunity also allowed me to join the Yorkville Volunteer Fire Department as a fully active member! Finally, I can mirror the dedication to our community that Mark Waterman had.

It was through two very special people, Todd and Sue Humiston, that I met the love of my life, Sarah, my best friend for life. In 1984, we married in a small church in Clayville, moved to Whitesboro, built our home, and joined the Whitesboro Volunteer Fire Department, the department where I still remain an active firefighter.

# 2

---

## My Firefighting Career Begins

As an active volunteer with Yorkville and Whitesboro, I was able to gain a great wealth of knowledge in fire tactics and leadership. I held many elected positions in both departments, culminating with the position of Chief of the Whitesboro department. Recently I served as their President and currently serve as the department Incident Safety Officer.

Never did I realize that the volunteer fire service would become my hobby and second love behind my wife and family. I was able to move through the ranks in various county associations and became President of the county volunteers as well as the county fire chiefs. On the state level, I serve as a Director for the Firemen's Association of the State of New York and Sergeant at Arms for the New York State Association of Fire Chiefs. In February of 2013, I was appointed a Deputy Fire Coordinator for Zone 1. In this position I was charged with planning and coordinating all of the fire training for the volunteers of Oneida County. While this can be challenging at times, it gives me a shot of energy each time I see young firefighters graduate from a New York State Firefighter 1 class. In 2014, I received my NYS Fire Investigator Level 1 certification and joined the Oneida County Origin and Cause team. I also sit as the Alternate Director for New York State to the National Volunteer Fire Council, a team very close to me since winning their Public Fire Educator of the Year Award in 1991. Thanks to this council, I was appointed to the NFFF Occupational Cancer Study Committee in hopes of improving the cancer issue in the volunteer fire service today. Also, I was appointed by Chief Kevin Quinn to serve as the NVFC's first Vice Chair of their Cancer Task Force with another Lymphoma survivor Chief James Seavey. So as you can see from this brief overview, I have so many opportunities to meet with danger through so many firematic opportunities. Never did I realize until being diagnosed with Non-Hodgkin B cell Lymphoma, that my "hobby" may kill me. What I loved to do best, helping others, just like Mark Waterman, would I ever think that I may never see my grand-kids, or travel south with my wife, or just sit around the station talking about the fire service. My life changed....and changed forever!

# 3

## WHAT WE DO AND DON'T KNOW ABOUT TODAY'S FIRES AND CANCER

Fires of today are so much different from the fires 15-20 years ago. Research proves that the fires in homes today are burning four times more BTU's than ever before. Today's fires grow at a much more rapid rate than yesterday's fires while exposing firefighters to significantly increased concentrations of highly carcinogenic agents. Today's residential fires have more carcinogenic materials in the building materials, furniture and electronic devices that if breathed or absorbed into the skin or lungs with proper care will develop an increase in cancer for that firefighter. What one time was a 15 minute escape time when the smoke detector goes off is now down to 3.5 minutes.

Research has shown that 56% of firefighters who died over the past few years according to the IAFF, died from cancer. This is an alarming statistics that seem to be growing into an epidemic around the fire service here in the United States. Multiple studies done by NIOSH demonstrated evidence and biologic creditability for statistically higher rates of multiple types of cancers in firefighters compared to the general American population including:

❈ Testicular cancer (2.02 times greater risk)
❈ Multiple myeloma (1.53 times greater risk)
❈ Non-Hodgkin's lymphoma (1.51 times greater risk)
❈ Skin cancer (1.39 times greater risk)
❈ Prostate cancer (1.28 times greater risk)
❈ Malignant melanoma (1.31 times great risk)
❈ Brain cancer (1.31 times greater risk)
❈ Colon cancer (1.21 times great risk)

✳ Leukemia (1.14 times greater risk)

✳ Breast cancer in women

Cancer has no bars or limits. Our skin temperature increases 400% for every 5 degree increase in body temperature. The use of self-contained breathing apparatus throughout the entire incident is crucial to a firefighters safety. Using proper decon procedures after the call and back at the station are an important part of the safety of firefighters. Deconing your apparatus following incidents as well. Toxic gases off-gas for approximately 72 hours after an incident. Developing sound practices so gear is not worn in the living quarters, or just stuck in the back of your SUV after incidents. The use of "baby wipes" or hand sanitizers on apparatus and at the station must be written into any safety practice in all departments. What we must recognize as a fire service is that cancer can be beat with early detections and screenings along with the support of your family, faith and the brotherhood.

# 4

---

## THE DIAGNOSIS

In November I went to my physician for a cold. Dr. Taylor informed me that I had swollen lymph node glands. I was provided with penicillin for 10 days, went on vacation with our friends, and found that the swollen glands went away. After two weeks the swelling came back and he suggested further evaluation from an Ear, Nose and Throat Specialist. So off to a new doctor named Dr. Obeid. After a brief examination of my nose and throat, he suggested a fine needle biopsy at St. Elizabeth's Hospital. On December 17th, when the test results came back Dr. Obeid informed us that I had B-Cell Non-Hodgkin's Lymphoma in the lower part of my left neck and tonsils area. That by far, was the worst day of our lives! It was further diagnosed as Stage II. That diagnosis really pulled the rug out from under us! In the words of Coach Jim Valvano, "Don't Give Up, Don't Ever Give Up" has become our motto from here on in! Jimmy, like me, never liked to lose, so we are planning our "attack" to beat this and become cancer free.

Thanks to our friends the Montana's, we were introduced to a teacher assistant from Westmoreland Road Elementary School (my old school that I was Principal at and where Ryan currently teaches) who shared with us the fact that we needed to get a second opinion and suggested Memorial Sloan Kettering Cancer Center (SK) in NYC. Her husband was treated there and has been cancer free for three years after being a Stage IV patient.

So we made an application to SK and heard back the very next day. Our experience with the registration process, the nurses, the doctors and the treatment we have received to date has been nothing short of first class! Sloan suggested that we have all pre-testing done here in Utica. You name it... and I've had the test... chest x-ray, CAT scan, PET scan, fine needle biopsy, open biopsy, bone marrow biopsy and NUMEROUS blood tests... the results confirmed the type of lymphoma but thankfully it did not show up in any other locations of my body... only in the lower part of my left neck and tonsils. That was some relief... as then it is considered "localized".

In January, we met with a Dr. M. Lia Polumba, a SK doctor that specializes just in lymphoma, she examined me, reviewed all the test results and suggested four options: radiation, a new FDA approved clinical trial, wait and see, or RCHOP (chemotherapy) therapy. She suggested that we meet with a Dr. Joachim Yahalom (Dr. Y), an internationally known radiation oncologist at Sloan and get his opinion. Dr. Y also teaches at the Cornell Med School in NYC.

For this first trip to SK was an experience to say the least! $300.00 for a hotel and $47 per day to park your car... we knew we weren't in Whitesboro anymore! We knew if we were in this for the long haul we needed to look into cheaper hotels and modes of transportation.

This past Monday we took the train from Albany and met with Dr. Y along with his oncology nurse and four other doctors. A much cheaper alternative! Dr. Y and his team studied my case for 2 hours before they came in to examine me. As they walked in, Dr. Y stated, "You are not as bad as we thought but...you are unique!" I said back to him, "Doctor, my wife tells me that daily!" He suggested that I undergo what is called, Intensified Modulated Radiation Therapy at SK. This is a computerized, 3-D type of radiation that focuses strictly on the lymphoma tissue and dissolves the cancer. He said that after the first week, you should feel the difference, and after 20 days, it should be gone from your body to never to come back again in that location.

OMG...finally some good news!!! This is a tiring process and they recommend that I bring a caregiver with me. So Sarah has a new title... caregiver!!!

Since this past Monday, Sarah has been like a travel agent. We were told to contact the American Cancer Society's Hope Lodge to see if they had availability. Their social worker who does the scheduling, informed us that they deal with 38 other New York/Long Island metropolitan area hospitals and that most of the rooms at the Hope Lodge are under renovation. So Plan B... through the wonders of the internet, Sarah found Staybridge Suites about five blocks from Penn Central where our train comes into. The subway from there to the hospital is at the end of our block so that makes it easy to get to and from the radiation sessions. They are giving us an AAA rate, plus it has a free breakfast in the morning, a full kitchen, laundry facilities and even receptions with finger foods. So we hope to get away with just the train, hotel, subway, and small meals.

We were called on Friday afternoon by Dr. Y's office and I have to meet with Dr. Kim, a SK dentist, on this Wednesday, he will be fitting me with a mouthpiece for the radiation sessions. I think Sarah may want to keep it after so she can keep my mouth shut! Then on Thursday I have to meet at 9:30 am with Dr. Y to prepare for the radiation, get the radiation tattoo on my neck and have the mask made for my face. This will be a three hour process and after that we will board the train back to Albany. We should know after Thursday when the radiation sessions will start. Hopefully sooner than later!

We will need to spend five days a week in NYC for 15-30 minute sessions each day. Our hope is that we can get a late Monday appointment so we can take the morning train in and an early Friday appointment so we can take the later train home, this saving weekend rates at the hotel. We will continue to use this blog to provide you with daily/weekly updates.

We want you to know that all your texts, emails, cards, phone calls and of course PRAYERS have not gone unnoticed. We truly believe "God is Good" and that he will guide us through this 'Bump in the Road!'

# 5

---

## ROUGH DAYS BEGIN

On Wednesday, February 5th, we had our pre-radiation appointment with the dentist at Sloan Kettering. With this early appointment and impending snow storm to hit the Northeast… we felt it best to travel to "The City" on Tuesday. Thank God we did!!! Trying to get around NYC with about 8" of snow on the ground, coupled with a rain and ice mixture… wasn't easy… and add in a suitcase in tow… walking was a challenge.

We saw it all today with chains on the bus tires, John Deere garden tractors plowing snow from the road and power brushes brushing the snow back into the road. Subways were delayed and forget hailing a taxi. Oh yes… the garbage was piled 5-6 feet high… no pick ups… the garbage trucks were used to plow the roads (see below)! (This makes you really appreciate the road care we experience from our Whitestown Highway and Whitesboro Village Transportation Teams!!!) Garbage trucks are used to plow the roads… but cars line the curbs and the plow isn't touching the pavement (I think it would help if they lowered it about 10 inches… don't you think?!) Garbage piles up due to the reappointment of these trucks!!! Gotta love NYC!!! But thanks to my "caregiver" Sarah, we made the appointment with time to spare. In fact, we went to noon mass at St. Patrick's Cathedral… Prayers are always good to have in your back pocket!

We met with a great dentistry staff at Sloan. I was brought in for a radial X-ray of my mouth ( I had to explain why I had so many sock threads in my mouth from Sarah stuffing socks in to shut me up)!!!

Honestly the dental team was awesome and we have the photos to bring back for Doc Konyak. After the X-ray, we met the dentists, Doctor Levi and Kim, who gave me the thumbs up… no mouthpiece required. Small victory!

On Thursday, February 6th we got up bright and early (oh yes… 7:00 am is early for retired educators)… we were to have my simulation today. We decided to check out of the hotel and take a taxi to Sloan Kettering (approx 3 miles away)... apparently 8:30 am is the height of commuter traffic... and everyone chose to take a taxi!!!! 45 minutes later in temps in the teens... we get a taxi to Sloan! We should have known then... that this wasn't going to be a great day. We had printed out the appointment schedule from Sloan's patient portal for our 10:00 am appointment... which we used to guide our preparations and appointment location for the day. The email sent us to the wrong building. Now Sloan is not a local hospital... it's six blocks long! Then we find out that Brian was supposed to fast for at least 6 hours prior to his PET Scan!!!!!!!!!!!!!!!!!!!! It wasn't on the patient portal, nor instructed when they called to inform us of this appointment. Needless to say... we were very disappointed! So back home we go!

We now have another appointment for Thursday, February 13th... for the simulation and PET Scan. Yes we will be fasting for this one! What happens in the simulation? They will be creating a mask for Brian to wear during his radiation treatments. This is a moist netting that covers his head and shoulders. As it dries... it molds to his face/shoulders.. and will prevent his head from moving during the radiation treatments. He also will get "Tatted Up"... a tiny tattoo on his left neck where the radiation will be focused. I asked them for a maltese cross tattoo, but not sure they appreciated that... LOL! We're learning more and more about the medical field as we take this journey to good health.

We will be leaving on Wednesday afternoon for NYC via car to Albany and train to NYC. If you have never traveled by train... especially to a busy metropolitan area... we highly recommend it. Comfy seats, free WiFi, no bridge tolls and no traffic hassles!

We cannot thank you enough for your cards, emails, texts, prayers, messages of support, medals, shamrocks, kind words and of course hugs. With your love and support... we will make this journey together.

But just remember... to my firefighters battling cancer....

"Don't Give Up. Don't ever give up" Jimmy Valvano

# 6

---

# THE SNOWPOCALYPSE (BRIAN'S DIAGNOSIS AND TREATMENT)

*Written Thursday, February 13th, 2014 by Sarah McQueen as the treatments began to impact Brian's health.*

As we sit in our NYC hotel room… We wanted to update you on Brian's "Road to Recovery". Due to our early appointment on Thursday, we travelled by car to Albany and then train to NYC. We are now staying in a different hotel… It is much closer to Sloan Kettering (located on East 48th street). Thanks to the generosity of Brian's brother Bob and other generous donations… most of the cost has been covered. Speaking of the McQueen Family… We were joined by our nephew Patrick (Bob's son)… For dinner and a very exciting Syracuse Game on the TV at The Perfect Pint, an Irish (bartender's were right off the boat!!!) bar/restaurant about 2 blocks from our hotel. Pat flew in from Boston, as he is helping to produce a segment for Good Morning America on Friday. He works for a company that helps business' with their charitable efforts. How exciting that game was… Ennis is the man!!!! We went to bed hearing that there was a chance of 4" of snow… And we woke to a blizzard and 10" of snow!! In our last post we told about the poor snow removal techniques… And nothing has changed. Our taxi's (we didn't want to chance the subway in weather like this) tires sputtered and spin… As the driver tried to drive up 2nd Ave!!! Garbage trucks… Three abreast pushed snow to the middle of the street… So God Bless the driver that had to change lanes! But we made it!!!! Brian's Appointment… Brian was prepared this time for the PET Scan and Simulation…. Fasting, no meds, no beverages other than water. They took him into the simulation room… And he emerged 3 1/2 hours later! He laid on a table and they placed a warm, moist plastic netting over his face and shoulders that dries quickly and becomes the mask he will wear for his radiation treatments. This is to make sure he is in the exact same position for each treatment. Brian was a trooper… No complaints from him… Personally I think the cute nurses had something to do with his smiles!!!

Appointment over… Back to the hotel… Its now raining and more snow is in the forecast! Side note to all our teacher friends… They had school today!!! The Mayor was deeply criticized for their decision and only 45% of the kids made it to school! Even in Central New York… Snow capital of the US… We cancel school under these circumstances. If you read or heard about Today Show Meteorologist AlRokers' rant over Twitter about the NYC Mayor…. Trust me he was 'spot on'!!!! Tonight we ventured out on foot to check out our new 'hood' and hopefully celebrate Valentine's Day. After burying our feet in 10"+ of snow, slush and ice… Multiple times we headed back to the hotel for dinner. They offer a free small buffet (burgers and salads) 2 nights/week at our hotel. It wasn't gourmet but it served its purpose. Back in our room to root on the U.S. Athletes… We find an email message… Our 11:20 am train back to Albany is cancelled due to the storm!!!! Yeah (with a lot of sarcasm)!!!! Oh no Brian says….Does this mean you will shop at Macy's again? We are now booked on the 5:47 train back to Albany! In the grand scheme of life… This is nothing! Updated Sunday, February 16th… We wanted to update everyone but couldn't send this out without adding some details about how we spent our Valentine's Day. The sun was out and since Brian and I didn't have to be on the train until 5:47pm we decided to walk around our new neighborhood. We found where there is a Sloan Kettering transit bus that goes from 53rd (5 blocks from our hotel) to the front door of SK. It leaves every 20 minutes… So taking a subway or taxi will be reserved for inclement weather days or "just not feeling the best" days. We also found a grocery store!!!! It sure isn't Price Chopper or Wegman's but we will be able to get food for small meals in our hotel room. Our room has a small kitchenette… Where I can be Betty Crocker. We also found several Irish establishments… Which makes us happy… It's always good to live around Lucky Irishmen!!!! So…. I did get a little shopping in at Macy's… With poor Brian towing the suitcase and wearing a backpack. He didn't make some New Yorkers happy when they got on the elevator with the suitcase…. I think Brian said something about needing an attitude adjustment!!!! We got to Penn Station around 1:30 pm with hopes of getting on an earlier train and after waiting online for 1 hour… We're told we can have 2 of the remaining 3 seats on the 3:15 pm train!!!! We're pumped!!!! We catch a quick sandwich at Garro's and head over to the "board" and see that the 3:15 pm is delayed!!!! So we wait….and wait…. And wait!!!! Two hours after the scheduled departure the train leaves Penn Station. We got into Albany around 8:00… Only to find 15" of snow on top of Brian's SUV…. And…. No snow brush!!!! Just another bump in the road! Home by 10:00… A clean driveway (thank you Ryan and Nick) and lots of mail! The cards and notes are wonderful….they keep us going. We love all of you!!!! Brian starts his treatments on Monday, February 24… And we will be be here for 4 weeks… 5 treatments per week. Home on Friday night… and back on Sunday. We can and will do this!!! We are fueled by your love and support. PS… As most of you know I like to take pictures…. I've started capturing photos to fit my theme "Only in New York City". I will share them with all of you when we celebrate Brian being cancer free! Love Sarah

# 7

---

## TREATMENTS BEGIN: THE ROAD TO RECOVERY

### Saturday, February 22, 2013:

While I attended the Verona Fire Department Installation Dinner, Sarah stayed home, packed and watched Syracuse lose to Duke (Jim I would have done the same thing!). While at the dinner, I spoke with Verona Fire Department Captain Rob Urtz who informed me last week that he was fighting Colorectal Cancer over the past year. Rob is an inspiration to me. He is undergoing both chemo and radiation treatments with a young wife and 2 children at home him. I gave him one of my lymphoma bracelets to wear and he showed me the one he got from an NFL coach who also was battling lymphoma. His outlook is very positive and just listening to his message; I realize that the time for me to beat this cancer is now. It's just amazing how many volunteer firefighters that I meet who have been impacted by cancer... all kinds of cancer. After that banquet, I picked up Sarah and off to the Barneveld FD Installation Banquet. While there I was able to thank both Chief Brian Healey and Captain Brian Palmer, who are working with Assistant Chief Brian DeStefanis of Deerfield FD, in creating a lime green lymphoma ribbon decal emblazoned with Believe 271 for firefighters' helmets. They will sell these decals, and use the proceeds to help other local firefighters, such as Rob, who are experiencing medical challenges. I say day in and day out, "There is no better brotherhood than what you find in the volunteer fire service."

### Sunday, February 23, 2013:

On Sunday, Sarah and I loaded up the car and off to Albany for our 12:15 Amtrak train to New York City. We have had some of the most memorable trips to NYC on the train. We arrived in NYC with a 41 degree temperature, grabbed a taxi, and oh what a ride it was! Taxi driver going 60 MPH down the street, stops to get change from his brother, and leaves the meter running!!! We reach our hotel just as Sarah starts to pull out her rosary! Our room, a gift from my brother, was super. It's large with a small kitchen set-up and quiet. My brother Bob has been amazing through all of this. Thank you both Bob and Nancy. Monday, February 24, 2013: Treatment Day 1 No one really knows what to expect when faced with your first treatment of radiation. I am no different, but having my wife as my rock to take each step with me made it so much better. We started with a great breakfast put on by our hotel. I can't say enough about the Residence Inn by Marriott on E. 48th Street. They have catered to all of our needs. At breakfast we were ready to put our thoughts together for what we know will be a trying experience.

Following breakfast we walked to St. Patrick's Cathedral to attend the noon mass. It is our intention to make this part of our daily routine, either before or after the radiation treatments. Following mass, we light a candle for my medical needs and one for our family and friends who have been there along the way. God has ridden my shoulder throughout this health issue, and I truly believe that it will be his guidance and your prayers that will get us through this. Thank you for being our angels.

Following mass we begin to walk to the MSKCC Outpatient office at 53 & 3rd street to catch the Sloan Kettering Shuttle. While walking over there we saw the sign for the FDNY Fire Store and with a few minutes to kill, stopped in there. (I hope you aren't surprised by this action.) Sarah and I met a retired FDNY firefighter named Ned Colter, whom we enjoyed talking to him about the fire service and fire prevention. He asked us both what our jobs were and why we were in New York. When I told him that on December 17, 2013, I was diagnosed with B-Cell Non-Hodgkin's Lymphoma, he said, "Why did you go to Sloan?" I explained to him that we were from Central New York and friends encouraged us to obtain a second opinion from Sloan. In fact one of the teacher assistants at Westmoreland Road Elementary School, Sue Bramhill, took her husband there with Stage 4 Cancer and he has been doing great for the past three years. Ned then informed us that he too was diagnosed with prostate cancer three years ago, went to Sloan, and has had a very good experience being cancer free for over two years. Sarah and I feel so great that no matter whom we run into, they have nothing but positive stories to tell us about their cancer treatment at Sloan. Speaking with Ned before my first radiation treatment really alleviated a lot of the nervousness that comes with not knowing what to expect.

We left the FDNY Fire Store and headed to the MSKCC Out Patient Center on 53rd Street where we were able to catch the shuttle. Upon entering Sloan, we were directed to the 4th floor where once again I had blood drawn for the radiation. Following that it was down to floor 2 and wait for the call. That came about 10 minutes later. I met the radiologist who will be working with me the next twenty treatments. She briefed me on the techniques that will be used, where the dressing room was located and introduced me to the team of professionals that will be providing the radiation treatments while here at Sloan. They were wonderful and helped to build my confidence as to what I should expect. Once in the room, I needed to approve the ugly photo of my face (with plastic netted mask) they took two weeks ago. "Yes, that's me." I'm reassured with the 'checks and balances' they use. Next comes the (said with sarcasm) attractive, comfortable mesh mask that is secured over my face then locked onto the table, x-rays follow, final size-up and the review by the physicist, who provides the final approval for first radiation treatment. Her words to the team were, "These are right on!"

Music to my ears! The team asked me if the music they were playing was good for me… it was boot stompin' country… so I approved. The radiation lasted 8-10 minutes and I didn't feel a thing. Before I knew it, it was over and I was sent on my way with the time schedule for my next four days in hand. As we leave Sloan via shuttle, one special memory sticks in my mind about the staff of Sloan.

When we sat down on the shuttle home, one person came on the bus and there were no seats remaining. An employee got up, asked the lady, "Are you a patient?" and when she answered yes, the employee got off the bus so the patient could ride this time. This exemplifies the caliber of workers that they have at Sloan. Patients care is #1. After returning to the hotel, I opened one of the twenty cards that were personally created by Betsy and Dan Schwertfeger. It was a photo card of Sarah and I dancing at Floyd's Installation Banquet, accompanied with the message, "You've gotta dance like there's nobody watching." After wiping the tears from my eyes, I looked to the ceiling and knew that God had something to do with this random act of kindness. After dinner at yet another Irish Restaurant (PJ Moran's on 48th), we head back to the hotel to watch Syracuse Basketball. We hear a knock on the door… and who has come to visit… Michelle Gibbs!!!! Whitesboro Class of 2009 and Syracuse Grad is living and teaching physical education in Zone 7, School 557 (don't quote me on the number) in New York. We had a great visit… I'm so proud of my former West Road student. I must say Chuck and Debbie you have one great daughter. So as I conclude this chapter, you'll be pleased to hear that we are more 'comfortable' living in the city… but we're definitely not ready to move here quite yet! Thank you for all your thoughts and prayers… you have no idea how much they mean to both of us.

# 8

## One Down and Three to Go

### Tuesday, February 25th / Treatment Day 2

We once again walked from the hotel to the MSKCC Outreach Center to obtain the shuttle off to the main campus for treatment 2. It was a brisk walk but refreshing and kind of provided me the opportunity to get focused on the treatments that will await me.

I checked in on the second floor and within minutes, my name was called and off to the changing room I go. Once dressed in the lovely gown, I was called into the same room as I had yesterday. I was introduced to two new members of the radiation team who were super with me. They checked my photo to make sure it was really me that was to get the noted treatment. In the background, there was classical (you know the elevator kind) music playing. I was asked by the radiologist what kind of music I wanted to listen to. My response was, "Not this crap!" OMG I thought the male radiologist wasn't going to stop laughing. They both turned to me and I said, "Top 40 or some country". They loved it? Once again the patient gets their wish and I was soon listening to Florida Georgia Line.

Next comes the infamous mask… Oh the mask!!! Mask on and locked to the table by the staff, they tell me this treatment wouldn't be as long as the first. They were correct! It was completed in 10 minutes. I'm thinking… "I can do this!"

Following the treatment we loaded onto the shuttle, with an awesome driver named Ian. These shuttle drivers take their acts of kindness right out of the Walt Disney employment book. They are just a wonderful group of people who make these trips so enjoyable. I think I only said, "Holy Crap", once on the trip back as a car pulled to within 1 inch of the side of our bus. (Sarah Edit: For those of you who really know Brian… insert an expletive for "Holy Crap!") Finally back to the clinic, walked home, stopped at the corner soup store and had lunch in our room.

One benefit of 'living' in the city… we get to connect with former students and friends… we don't get to see in Central New York. Tonight was one of those opportunities! Richard Krouse (aka 'Rock the House Krouse'), Oriskany Class of 1992, met us for dinner at Tony Di

Napoli's in Times Square. Richard is now the head equipment manager for the New York Islanders. He always loved hockey.... Starting with the Utica Devils... and now is in his dream job. As Richard says, "Life's Swell in the NHL!"

On Wednesday, Michael Geller... a fellow school board member and good friend, treated us to dinner. He was in the city on business. The food was amazing and we enjoyed it a second time in the form of leftovers on Thursday. It's such a treat to connect with friends from the 'Boro while we're here.

### Thursday, February 27th / Treatment 4:

It was a great day for all of us. Following the radiation, I had to have a follow-up appointment with the oncologists (Yahalom and Yang) that designed my personalized IMRT program. They both evaluated my progress and were very impressed with the downsizing of the cancer in my neck. Their comment was, "You're right where we want you to be." That put a smile on both of our faces. Treatment 5 was our last treatment for the week. We arrived at the hospital earlier than usual and within five minutes I was taken into the changing room to prep for the fifth day. As I walked into the radiation room a smile came across the two radiologists... they were happy knowing that they could listen to music that they could appreciate (apologies to those classical musical lovers). I have a great team of radiologists and I have SO MUCH respect for anyone in that position. Following the treatment we headed to the train station for our train back to 'reality' and our wonderful community of Whitesboro and Oneida County. God it was great to see Ryan, Erin, my brother Bob and so many friends who have provided me with peace of mind and the will to continue. While at home, I found out about a brother firefighter and paramedic from the Schuyler Fire Department and Kunkel Ambulance who was recently diagnosed with colon cancer. His name is Anthony Pagliaro (Pags). He, as well, will be on his way to Sloan for a second opinion leaving Sunday for a Monday appointment. Our thoughts and prayers are with Pags and his family. March 2nd / Week 2: We drive to Albany and back on the 12:15 pm Amtrak train to the city. It was great that I was able to Facebook with Pags on the way down and reassure him that he is going to the right place for his second opinion. I hope to see him there but not promising since the hospital covers six blocks! Here we are back at the Residence Inn in the same room that we had last week (our request... but their attention to providing the best for their guests)! We unpacked, more clothes than we take to a cruise vacation... really Sarah do you need 5 pairs of shoes and boots!!! We walked to St. Patrick's Cathedral for the 5:30 pm Mass, where we lit a candle for Grandma Cichon, Mrs. Head, Pags and myself. God is great and anytime that I can talk with Him inside His own house gives me a positive outlook. Following Mass, Sarah and I went to Bob's Burger Bar for a quick bite to eat. Once we paid the bill, Sarah, in one of her most graceful moves putting on her coat, swept by the vinegar bottle and proceeded to send it crashing to the floor and all over the people that were sitting next to us. (Sarah Edit: "I was trying one of those Lutz' that Courtney Gouger and Hannah Kulik can do on ice!") At that time I ran out of the restaurant not wanting to pay another bill and we walked home.

In closing, .TRUST ME... this is no vacation.... But the outcome should be a cancer free life....

March 3rd, Monday Today is the coldest day since we've been here. As we walk to the shuttle, the wind and bitter cold just seeps through our coats. My schedule is provided to me on Friday and all of my times this week are at 12:30pm. Every Monday, the team takes additional X-rays to see if the program from the previous week needed to be changed. This means that I am in the mask for about 20-25 minutes. Not my most favorite part of this treatment but after the x-rays, the team said the pictures looked good and they were ready to continue with the radiation. 6 down and 14 to go!!!! Following our treatment we loaded back on the shuttle, stopped for a deli sandwich, chips and a cookie... $42.00 latter we were out the door! Boy do we miss those prices at Charlie's Pizza in Whitesboro.

Sarah and I are just hanging out here at the hotel to continue our updates for you. We were surprised with mail... yes... mail! We got a funny card from our favorite nurse and Carla from "The Road". We are blessed!

# 9

---

## FROZEN IN NYC

### Tuesday, March 4th: Week #2, Day #2

It's another cold and windy day in NYC. Sarah and I walked to the 53rd street shuttle once again and the brisk air was refreshing. Once on the shuttle, it gave me time to really reflect of some of the things that I have learned about cancer. Cancer can affect anyone… From young, old, male, female, small children, every color, race and creed… cancer has seeped into our lives. Seeing some of these cancer patients brings tears to my eyes. It makes me realize what a great support team will see me through this. Every day since being diagnosed, I wear the bag of soil attached to a chain that is from Saint Mother Marianne's grave. It was given to me by Sister Dolorosa Lenk, my aunt. I wear it in hopes of becoming the next miracle become cancer free. Utica Football Coach Blaise Faggiano sent me a St. Blaise medal and prayer that has been around my neck since my diagnosis. It hangs on a chain right next to my St. Florian medal. The Beck Family, Erin and Chris gave me an Irish Blessing Cross that I keep in my pocket daily. These will never leave me as I know the meaning behind each of them and what they mean to Sarah and me.

The twenty cards that Betsy and Dan Schwertfeger made for me to open after each treatment… bring both a tear and a laugh to us as we read the personal message written on the inside. Finally, the phone calls to "check in" from our 'favorite' son and daughter in law. All are truly messages from the heart! All of these "personal" messages and gifts are what are getting me through this treatment. The constant texts, emails and calls from our close friends and family back home. The fire service support that I have received from all across the county has made this medical healing process so much better. Calls from my mother-in-law a few times a week, telling me that she prays for me daily, means so much to me.

The constant encouragement on Facebook and the Believe 271 campaign that Barneveld FD is doing that will help others like me and their families in the future. Just today I received a boost in an email from Justin Gorski, a graduate of Whitesboro whom I coached in Biddy Basketball. He said, "Mr. McQueen, it's time to fight like a Warrior, just like you told us to do when we beat the Spartans. You will beat cancer." How proud I was to read he's found his love of his life and is getting married next year. He is working as a Sports Information Director of a baseball team in Oklahoma. God has blessed me with a wonderful family, great friends and the courage to tackle what lies ahead.

Today I gutted the infamous mask out without the medicine. All went well and in 15 minutes I was back out and ready to do our walk for the day. So we attempt to walk to the AAA in NYC, nine blocks away. We only made it five as the chill just ran through our bones. So my tour director, Sarah, says let's go to a movie matinee. So we did. We saw a great movie called "Non-Stop." Have you ever been to an afternoon matinee in NYC? Well the movie was $29.00 and the small diet coke and small bag of popcorn was $13.00. I think I took stock out in the wrong company. Following the movie we grabbed dinner at a deli and brought it back to our hotel. Yup...in NYC...and no SU game on...but there is "Chicago Fire!"

### Wednesday, March 5th: Week #2, Day #3

Rough night last night! Throat getting a little sore, but nothing I can't deal with. I checked my email before I left... and what do I find? ...but yet another picture of someone wearing a "No One Fights Alone" bracelet is sent to us. The bracelet photos from West Road School we have received over the last two weeks mean the world to us... thank you for sharing!
Thank You to my Westmoreland Road...aka..."The Road"
Teachers...you mean the world to me!

Off to the hospital on a day that shows promising spring weather in NYC. Temperature at 38...heat wave! Made it to Sloan for the radiation, same team greeted me, and they even took me in a little early. All went well so 8 down and 12 to go! Sarah tells me... "You're more than 1/3 done!" She loves math... and all these fractions make me think she's baking! After the shuttle ride back, we embarked on our 7 block walk to St. Patrick's Cathedral for 12:30 mass and ashes. Always feel better walking out of St. Patrick's! Following mass and ashes we did our walk around the Plaza, stopped at Lenny's Deli (highly recommended by Sue Bramhill) and then back to the hotel. Our pedometers are working overtime as we are trying to put 3-5 miles a day on walking. Once back to the hotel we found a card from our Remsen friends, Robert and Melissa Eaton and their children on our table. So nice to know that people care and show it in so many ways. Then the infamous Betsy Card...today it was the photo from the Tunnel to Tower Run/Walk from last year with the quote, "Life is like a rollercoaster, you can either scream every time there is a bump, or you can throw your hands up and enjoy the ride." Our goal is to enjoy the remaining 12 days of this ride in hopes that God has a plan for me to be cancer free!

### Wednesday, March 6, 2014: Week #2, Day #4

Today is Doctor Day! So Sarah and I left a little early as today is the day I have to give blood, take my radiation and then see the doctor. All went well today...but OMG...it was so cold again. Like in CNY it was in the high teens and low 20's but the wind chill made it feel like the coldest day since we have been here. (I think we've said that before... but who goes for a 3-4 mile walk in single digits?!)

We arrived early at the Main Hospital, checked in and were told, don't get comfortable it was time to go in and get the treatments. So off I went to meet my outstanding radiation team. I am definitely stopping at Holland Farms to bring them in some CNY treats for Monday. All went well with the treatment, so I left, went to get my blood work and then off to see Dr. Yahalom. His nurse, Kathy, came in first and checked to see how things were going. My throat and back of my mouth have become a little sore so she prescribed a mouthwash for the discomfort. Due to the discomfort I had to change my eating habits and have to eat "soft, non-spicy" foods that will not irritate my throat and mouth. Oh well… I always wanted to lose weight so started on this new "diet" this past Tuesday and Sarah says she has noticed a difference already. Dr. Yahalom came in and put me on his examination table. He felt my neck, looked at his nurse and said, "What side of his neck had the issue?" At first I didn't know how to take that, but knew he was kidding and was impressed that he realized that the cancer was diminishing. This always makes me feel great and reaffirms the fact that I am in the right place. In fact he spoke about reviewing the program and changing the radiation dosage and will talk more about it this on Monday with us. Following the hospital visit, we returned to the hotel, got off the shuttle hallway back, and got our walk in for the day. We are hopeful that next week will be warmer and we won't have to wear 2 layers under our winter coats, plus scarves, hat and gloves.

Thanks again for all the pictures, texts, phone calls, prayers and emails… they keep us going. Tomorrow we will celebrate being "Halfway to the Cure!"

# 10

THE PAIN BEGINS...AND SO DOES BELIEVE 271

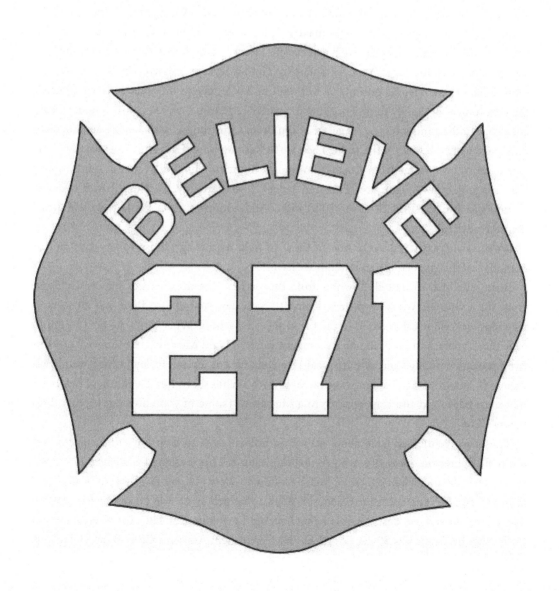

## Friday, March 7th: Week #2, Treatment Day #10

*NOTE: This part is written by Sarah… due to the increase in pain of my treatment plan.*

Friday means… pack up and head for "Home Sweet Home" after Brian's 12:30 treatment is complete. Brian's throat and mouth are beginning to exhibit soreness but the thought of going home overrides any pain he may be experiencing. (Could the man that loves to go on vacation be wishing he was home… you bet!!!). Sitting in the waiting room with a room packed full of cancer patients also waiting for their treatments… makes us closely watch the minute hand on our watches. Brian's 12:30 appointment slot comes and goes… and he still hasn't entered the treatment room. Finally at 1:15 one of the perennial upbeat receptionists Rob, calls out "McQueen".… We look at each other and say "We're going to miss our 2:20 train!" I reassure Brian that we might make it (I knew we wouldn't). He exits the treatment and skips the \*mouth car wash (we'll explain this later)… with hopes that we can make it to the train. No such luck… as Maxwell Smart (of Get Smart) we "missed it by that much!" 10 minutes late… train leaves on time… without out 2 McQueen's on board! We try to catch the next train at 3:15 only to find out that it cost $66.20 extra… you know rush hour… take advantage of the commuters… we get it! I calm Brian's frustrations with a delicious chocolate milkshake while we wait for the train. Then we're "Home Sweet Home" at 7:30 pm. Yes, "Air Brian" drove from home from Albany!! We come home to a bin full of mail… cards, notes, homemade goodies (thank you Tina and Janet)… we certainly are blessed with the best friends and family EVER!!!! Over 100 cards…And counting…you know truly who your friends really are!

We're saving each and every one of these to help us through those tough days and to remind us of the great family and friends we have!!!

Brian says "that it went all downhill from this point!" The dreaded side effects decide to come for a visit and overstay their welcome!!!! Saturday, March 8th: Brian has all sorts of meetings and phone calls related to the fire service and school. What would he do if he didn't have these hobbies to keep him busy… maybe dust?!?! Nah! Me either!!! He meets up with two fire service buddies out of Barneveld Fire Department, Brian Healey (Chief) and Brian Palmer (Captain). Brian Palmer was a member of the Whitesboro Fire Department before he moved to Barneveld and is married to Mia Massarotti (some of you know her brother, firefighter George F.).

These two gentlemen have come up with a brilliant idea to help out other current and future firefighters in our region who are battling cancer. They designed a "Believe 271"decal that can be added to a helmet, car or home window to show our common goal of beating this crippling disease. The cost of each decal is $5.00, of which 100% will go to this foundation. There are no overhead costs, as it is being handled by volunteers. The cost of creating and producing the decals was $0.00. Deerfield Fire Department Assistant Chief Brian DeStefanis generously donated his graphic time and covered the cost of materials. The Brotherhood is very strong is Central New York.

What is Believe 271? Those of you who are a volunteer firefighter in Oneida County already know... but for the rest of you... here is the explanation. Brian is one of four Deputy Fire Coordinator's for Oneida County. His "call" number is 271. Ok... you got it now!!!

We were sent pictures of the 271 Believe decals in use...

Brian's Car 271 Helmet.....Sauquoit VFD.....Oriskany VFD....Barneveld Chief Brian Healey....Westmoreland Past Chief Brad White....Barneveld Captain Brian Palmer.....Oriskany Fire Chief Jeff Burkhart....Verona Captain Kevin Oatman....Holland Patent Fire Chief Dan Kalk....Polk County Lt. (Nephew) Joe McQueen....Oriskany / Whitesboro Central School, "Chick Clique' Theresa Kozien, Terri Sojda, Sue McBain, me, Ellen Tuttle

The pictures of your... Believe 271 Helmet Decals and the No One Fight's Alone Bracelets were so important to meet the pain and suffering Brian was having.

Saturday night we were going to attend the play at the Middle School, Annie Jr., but those plans were changed as the painful symptoms of throat/neck radiation became quite evident to Brian. Sunday, March 9th: We take our usual train out of Albany and arrive in a chilly but bearable New York at 3:00 pm. We lost an hour of sleep last night due to Daylight Savings... but it's so nice to have that extra hour of sunshine! The way Brian was feeling made the two hour train ride feel like a lot more. I let Brian rest... and I head out by myself (getting brave) to go to the grocery store, Morton Williams on 2nd Avenue. This grocery store is about the size of McDonald's (minus the Play Space)! It has the most bizarre aisles... about 3 feet wide... only 1 cart width and is just a little pricey!!! Below are pics of 2 of my purchases. A can of Campbell's soup and 4 butter pats (I didn't want to buy a whole pound... to make Brian his favorite grilled cheese sandwich). Then one of those moments when you know you're not in Kansas anymore... on my walk back to the hotel... I see Rodent Repellent Garbage Bags filled at the curb. How encouraging to know that the mice, rats, and raccoons can't get into the neighbor's garbage. (This one's for you Betsy... maybe the establishments near O'Hara's could use these...lol) Brian is beginning to suffer from extreme mouth and throat pain... we try everything to alleviate the pain... gargle, sprays, aspirin... even Orajel... and nothing helps! He can't even talk... hmmm... is this a bad thing? Sorry Brian... I couldn't miss the opportunity to pick on you when you can't respond! It was truly a painful night in the hotel. Brian would sleep 30 minutes, waking up to the pain and phlegm that has gathered in his mouth. Try to take care of it and try to fall back to sleep... not much success! Monday, March 10th:

### Week #3, Treatment Day #11

*From Brian's perspective*... and of course edited by the detailed Sarah (Ms. OCD)! After a not so good sleeping night, we thought we'd head to the hospital sooner to see if we could see Cathy the oncologist's nurse. Sarah sent her a detailed message of the severe pain that I was going through the night before. Cathy saw that my mouth had some significant sores in it and that I would need to take a mouth wash treatment (aka *mouth car wash) after each radiation. They knew the pain was intense when they gave me the old, "What's the pain level from 1-10 with 10 being the worst. I mumble... 10!!!" Hence, they provided me with oxycodone to help with the pain. What is a *Mouth Car Wash? Imagine a mini car wash sprayer hooked up to a saline (salt water) solution and used to continuously spray in the mouth, under the tongue and down the throat. After radiation we see Dr. Yahalom who was impressed with the treatments so far. Sarah asked if we are still on target for the 20 days of treatment and he said "Yes." We can only hope and pray. On Monday, the pain meds are doing their job and I take a 2 ½ hour nap... and Sarah makes me a gourmet (Sarah edit) Toasted Cheese Sandwich. Followed up with applesauce. Social Media... love it or hate it... it has been our saving grace!!!! We have been able to connect with so many friends and family... and former students!!! Tonight we heard from Philip Melkun, Tracy O'Connor Day and Missy Loftus... great people. We are blessed to have you praying for Brian... God Bless! This evening the pain was lessened but the mouth sores were still quite evident. Once again I had a sleepless night.

**Tuesday, March 11th: Week #3, Treatment #12**

We took the shuttle to the hospital in hopes of getting an early treatment with the mouth car wash. Nope... that didn't work out. They took me right in for the radiation treatment. At that time my team told me that this soreness will stay around for about 2-3 weeks after the last treatment on March 21st. Great! I was thrilled to hear that.....NOT! Following the treatment I went over for the mouth car wash once again. There a new nurse spotted some sores in my mouth that she believes would be better served with the famed "Magic Mouthwash." They will prescribe it and I can pick it up tomorrow. It was such a nice day with temps in the 60's; I went back to the hotel room to deal with this pain.

I encouraged Sarah to take a break as nurse/maid and go visit the Guggenheim Museum. Her college roommate and current art teacher at Minisink Valley, Roberta, said this was the museum to visit while in NYC. Good choice Roberta... she really enjoyed the Carrie Mae Weems Photography Exhibit... and would recommend it to others. (Sarah Edit) A side note about Roberta... if it wasn't for Roberta... Brian and I wouldn't be married today. Oriskany Teachers and Retirees will appreciate this story. Roberta grew up in the Poughkeepsie area, was my roomie at Oneonta, student taught in Oriskany (with Mary McCullough)... living in an apartment inside the current Kernan Law Offices... and landed a job teaching 3rd grade at Oriskany in the fall of 1977. I was hired to teach at the Oriskany High School. Then about 1 week before school was to start (1978), she resigned and moved closer to her husband's new place of employment. Guess who gets hired.... The three piece suit man... Brian McQueen. There is more to the story about who is responsible for our dating... but I'll save that to another time.

I'm rested and ready to watch "The Best Darn TV Show".... Chicago Fire... and they did not disappoint! I fall asleep at 11:15 pm only to be shocked out of sleep at 12:45 am by the fire alarm. Yes, "the boys" from the firehouse on 51st street show up with Engine #8, Ladder #2 and Battalion #8... only to find out it was a false alarm. Thank Goodness!!! Wednesday,

March 12th: Week #3, Treatment #12 Around 9:30 am we awaken to multiple sirens... and already TJ Ryan has text me about an explosion in the city (does he have the scanner from every city on his phone?)! We are about 60 blocks south of the explosion but the impact of the blast and story is felt in Midtown Manhattan. We instantly think of Greg Williams, from Clinton (NY), who works out of the NYFD firehouse on 133rd street! I was scheduled to do my 'ride along' with Greg today! We text Greg and tell him to Stay Safe... as we guess he is involved in the explosion incident. We also ask him to delay my 'ride along' until next week when hopefully I will feel better.

I experienced another very restless night due to the soreness in the mouth and throat; we headed back to the hospital in hopes of finding better answers. I went in for my radiation and of course this team was so kind and caring. I really love this team! They tell you the way it is, and that's what I wanted to hear. After the treatment we waited a while to get the mouth car wash. I had a new nurse do the wash today, Melissa, and she was the best yet. She realized that I had infections in my mouth that needed medical treatment through a pill. She didn't waste any time as she went right to Dr. Yahaloms' assistant, Dr. Lanning, brought him in, and his words were. "OH YA YOU ARE RIGHT, its Thrush!" He told us that he had prescribed, Fluconazole, and that we could pick it up in an hour at their pharmacy downstairs. I could have given Melissa a hug, as she didn't just do the mouth car wash, she recognized the issue and addressed it. She's not as good as Super Nurse Wendy Karas... but a close wanna be! Around 2:30 pm we hear from Greg Williams... he's safe... and yes he was at the explosion and will extend my ride along invite until next week.

So, as we leave the hospital and shuttle back to the hotel, we hear about the freezing rain and lousy conditions forecast for tomorrow. But, not nearly as bad as the CNY people are getting! Ryan and Erin check in nightly and tells us of the 8" of snow on the ground already with another 4-8" yet to come. As we returned to the hotel, we had three cards waiting for us from our friends. One was from two of my favorite "West Roaders", Carla Ryan and Wendy "Doc" Karas. These two people are some of the reasons why Westmoreland Road Elementary School is the Best! The other cards are from our Melissa, Bob, Devin and Skylar Eaton who sent us a card last week, too. Melissa, you must have picked out the card... it's perfect to what I wanted to say to the nurse! AND of course Dan and Betsy's daily card, opened every day after completion of my radiation treatment. It is through these random acts of kindness, very similar to the receiving of cards, texts and emails, that is allowing me to Stay Strong through this painful time of the treatment, I realize that no matter how much it hurts now, one day I'll look back and realize it changed my life for the better. Thanks again for all the pictures, texts, phone calls, prayers and emails... they keep us going. On Friday, we will celebrate being "Three-Fourths Way to the Cure!" God Bless and Hugs from both of us, Brian and Sarah

# 11

---

## NEARING THE END OF TREATMENTS

### *NOTE: This has been written by Brian and Sarah...*

#### Friday, March 14th: Week #3, Treatment Day 15

Time to celebrate... we are officially ¾ or 75% complete!!!!
After the treatment, we grab our luggage and a taxi and head to Penn Station. We must look like we know what we're doing. We've had people stop us and ask us for the location of the closest subway and which one to take. I do hope they aren't still riding on the subway we suggested without finding their intended destination!

No delays on the train, no snow on the car in Albany... its smooth sailing home! I run off to meet Sue McBain (a former colleague and dear friend) at Oriskany High School. They are putting on the musical, "Bye, Bye Birdie". What a fantastic job the cast, crew and directors (2 new teachers) did with this production. I was very impressed with the acting and singing. I think they haven't done a musical since 1975 (before I started teaching there....I know... and most of you weren't born yet)! When I get home at 10:00, Brian is deep in sleep!

#### Saturday, March 15th:

We open the tons of mail we get over the week... and are warmed by the numerous cards we get from members of the Whitesboro community, former colleagues, fire service associates, family and friends. I said this before... "It's the fuel that keeps us going!"

Brian finds solitude in 'going to the firehouse'. How many times have I told people on the phone when they call for Brian... "He's at the firehouse.... His second home." I guess I never realized how strong that bond was until we were faced with this challenge. The fire service has been there through the good and bad, supporting us in our time of need and celebrating with us (and oh boy do they know how to celebrate!) when it was warranted. They truly are the best brother and sisterhood!!!

For the first time in five years, we watch the Utica St. Patrick's Day Parade on TV. We've always had a great time walking or riding on the Massarotti Family Float in the parade...

throwing beads and sharing Debbie Gibbs' Leprechaun Pudding Shots. We'll be back next year... "Bigger and Better!"

Saturday night we are treated to Game Night at Ryan and Erin's home. After getting beat in the "Game of Life" and "Scattergories"... we head home to pack for hopefully our last trip to NYC. Brian is so sick of packing and living out of a suitcase he wants me to sell our suitcases in the garage sale. How do people like his brother Bob do this weekly?!

**Sunday, March 16th:**

Our usual routine commences for the 4th time... leave by 10:00, drive to Albany, train to New York, and check in by 4:00. Yada, yada, yada....

They put us in a different room for the first time in 4 weeks... I'm nervous that I will try to get into our old room number (that only happened once... lol... not bad!). I look out our window at the condos across the street and discover a roof top playground and 'picnic' area (see picture below). City kids grow up so differently than those in our neck of the woods. Brian heads off to 5:30 mass at St. Patrick's Cathedral. He lights candles for Gordy and Colleen Kotars, Mike Whelan and Anthony Pagliaro.

I have been invited by Pam Graniero (Paula Flisnik's sister) to see her daughter Nicole ballet dance in a production at NYU called "Stories from the Night Before". Nicole dances for the American Ballet Theater and is my daughter-in-law's (Erin) cousin. Nicole was amazing... what poise and elegant to her dance.

**Monday, March 17th: Week #4, Treatment Day #16**

Could it be? The last week of radiation?!?!?!?!?! Top 'O the Mornin' to you... it's Happy St. Paddy's Day!!! We want to express our gratitude to the doctors, nurses and staff at Sloan Kettering with a gift from Central New York. So we brought them 2 dozen half moon cookies from Holland Farms. They loved them!!!! Riding back from the hospital on the shuttle bus to 53rd street, I begin to notice more and more Irish 'establishments' decked out in their green, orange and white. This is a town that surely knows how to celebrate St. Patrick's Day. You would be a rich man if you could collect all the money from the recyclables. The weather is bitter cold and we can't wait to get back to our room. We watch the NYC St. Patrick's Day Parade from the comfort of our hotel room. Naptime for Brian! Later on we decide to venture out in search of a hearty soup for dinner. We find ourselves following (maybe chasing) a ladder truck from the Fire Station on 51st street. When you live in the city, hearing a fire siren is a common sound. We get a phone call from my former boss, Andy Brown and messages from several former Oriskany students. I had to smile at the comment from one... Derek Gorski... now a doctor at Syracuse Upstate Medical (so proud of him)... he stated, "You know, Brian used to offer us McDonald's gift certificates to take a charge... I feel like we should be giving them back now!" Oh how Brian loved coaching... he misses it... and yes a good portion of his salary went to team pizza parties or Mickey D's certificates... anything to motivate the team.

**From Brian...** What a surprise? I received a text from an Oriskany alumnus (Class of 1990 I think), Mike Trinkaus, who also played sports for me in 'Otown'. Good friend and fellow basketball coach Mike Deuel made contact with him. Deuel and I took Trink to 5 Star Basketball Camp in Pennsylvania prior to his senior year. Mike was just a great kid. He was a pure shooting forward and worked hard on the court and in the classroom. He went on to SUNY Brockport majoring in accounting and got his MBA at Fordham University. Today he is a financial planner in Connecticut and doing very well. He heard about my medical issue and emailed us two tickets to the Knicks-Pacers game for this Wednesday evening. What a class act! But that is Mike Trinkaus. You never know how many lives you've impacted, not having seen Mike since he left for college; it kind of makes your day! Thanks for the hook-up Coach D!

**Tuesday, March 18th: Week #4, Treatment Day #17**

When will the cold ever end... another bitterly cold day! Cathy Adams, Dr. Yahalom's nurse, comes out to the waiting room to greet Brian. She thanks him for the Half Moon Cookies and says that he is "on target" to be finished with his radiation treatments on Friday. It's great to see Brian smile!

We take our familiar walk to St. Patrick's Cathedral to attend mass and light candles. Today they are for Mary Hitchcock's husband (Frank), Rich Riley and Andy Brown's sister-in-law (Mary Ann). We know that God has been with us on this journey and have asked him to look out for our friends.

I drag Brian to Macy's for a little retail therapy... he's a good sport... he'd rather be sleeping! Brian has found that the radiation treatments are sucking the energy right out of him. He naps almost every afternoon now. His skin has reddened; he has a nasty cough and skin dryness. I try my best to care for his skin and cough.

On the news they mention that the Mega Million Lottery is around 400 million... so I run out in search of a ticket... because "Hey You Never Know!" This isn't an easy task... after about 2 mile hike... I find a location. (p.s. I won.... $1.00!!!)

Brian is contacted by Brian Healey, Barneveld's Fire Chief. He is relaying the latest numbers on the Believe 271 decal efforts. We reported on this in an earlier chapter. Basically it's an effort to raise funds to help other firefighters who are afflicted with cancer. The response has been overwhelming. The original goal... started on March 8th, was to raise $5000.00. They have already met and exceeded that goal. No firefighter will ever fight cancer alone again!

It's Tuesday night... so that means "Chicago Fire" on TV!

**Wednesday, March 18th: Week #4, Treatment Day #18** We're "rounding third and heading for home"!!!!! We come back to our hotel right after treatment with a hearty soup in hand. Brian tries eating a blueberry muffin... but the flavor and texture stop him in his tracks. He's losing weight and tells me he will be wearing a Speedo by the pool this summer. We walk in our room to find we have mail... who gets mail in NYC... in a hotel? It's another card from the Bob and Melissa Eaton (Remsen Fire Chief) and family. Brian opens one of his last 3 cards from the Schwertfeger's. This one includes a picture of me snorkeling in the Caribbean last November. Brian laughs hysterically... that is a great story... ask him about it! Ryan and

Erin make their daily phone call. We are blessed to have them in our lives. They are the BEST kids a parent can have. Brian naps most of the afternoon. He has to rest up for a big night... Knicks Basketball!!! We arrive at the game via taxi... he must have thought we wanted a tour, too... he takes us down 5th avenue which is bumper to bumper with taxi's... $21.00 later we join hundreds of others trying to get into Madison Square Garden. Phil Jackson and several celebrities (Matthew Morrison – Glee, Olivia Wilde, Edward Burns... but no Spike Lee) are at the game. It's a great night for Melo and the Knicks... they beat the Pacers 92-86. Thank you Michael Trinkaus... that was a dream come true for us. When we get home... we are messaged a picture from Erin's sister, Dr. Laura Flisnik (Georgetown University)... she shows her support of Brian with a Lymphoma pin on her work uniform. We get a great call from our nephew Pat from Boston and Tina Passalacqua (aka Mrs. P) sends us pictures of her granddaughter Avery wearing the "No One Fights Alone" bracelet. We feel the love and support!

### Thursday, March 19th: Week #4, Treatment Day #19

It's a big day... treatment, mouth wash... and see the oncologist for the last time! We do our usual walk to 53rd street. That is the outpatient hospital for Sloan and where you will find a great human being. His name is Pete. He's become our friend over these four weeks. Why is he so special? ...Because the patient is always #1. We find a lot of the staff at Sloan has these same qualities but Pete rises above the others. We thank him for what he does and you can tell he's humbled by Brian's words. Brian has a little extra energy in his step today... his next to last treatment and mouth wash... who wouldn't?! We meet with Cathy Adams, oncologist nurse, and Dr. Rimner (filling in for Dr. Yahalom). Both say everything is on target. The dry, redness of his skin will improve over time. I think there was a hint there that his nurse Sarah needs to apply the medicated cream more often. He shares his lack of appetite and taste for food... so Cathy decides to weigh Brian. He has lost almost 20 pounds! This isn't the diet he wanted to go on though. Dr. Rimner says that Dr. Yahalom will want to see Brian again 4-6 weeks from now. They will repeat the PET Scan, he'll meet with the dentist and have a full exam. They will be able to tell them how successful the radiation was. So we will have to wait again... ugh!!! However we believe our faith and friends will guide us to a cancer free report! We come home (what am I saying... it's not home... it's the hotel) and find 2 cards from Angels Wendy Karas and Carla Ryan... how thoughtful they are. Brian opens a Betsy created Schwertfeger card that has another picture from our Cancun trip... oh! I wish we were there.

Time to get ready for the Syracuse vs. Western Michigan NCAA game... I get Brian all relaxed... and he falls asleep! He wakes up just in time to catch much of the last four minutes. Good Job 'Cuse!!!!

This is it for this Chapter... tomorrow we will head back HOME!!!!! We truly appreciated your love; support and generosity are we handled this 'bump in the road'. It was you that got us through those tough days, moments. Your cards, texts, messages, phone calls, cards, donations, and most of all... hugs that has carried us along this journey. We owe all of you huge hugs and kisses!

# 12

---

## Where Do We Go From Here

Thank you for allowing me to share my trials and tribulations with you. Let's take a look at where we need to be as firefighters. Some great discussion enclosed with hopes of actions taken by those who wear the bugles in your department. We need a team effort to change the culture of the fire service today.

The need to embed solid firefighter safety measures in all departments' Best Practices is a must. Early education to the dangers of cancer in the fire service should be included in all probationary firefighter training. Educating our younger firefighters to the dangers that they will face in the future will allow them to build a better foundation of safety. By starting at an early age our new recruits will realize that there is a new badge of courage portrayed through their eyes.

As fire service leadership, we need to change the culture of the fire service. We need to walk the talk and lead by example. It's not good to wear black soot on your face, helmet and gear. The same goes for your hoods. Make it mandatory to wash your hoods after every major fire and/or once a week. Sit down with your elected officials and discuss the need for a spare set of gear, hoods and helmets. We can have all the recruiting programs in the world, but whats good does it do if we don't retain them through a positive health and wellness safety program?

To my firefighters stricken with cancer, and to those whose families, walk along side them. You are the inspiration for us all! Cancer can be beat! If you think of it as you think of firefighting, you can't do it alone. When that doctor tells you: "You Have Cancer," while you think of the worst, you need to think of those who have battled and won the fight in front of you.

There are so many resources in the field today that will provide you with information. The Firefighters Cancer Support Network, Firemen's Association of the State of New York, New

York State Association of Fire Chiefs, National Volunteer Fire Council and the National Fallen Firefighters Foundation are just a few resources on a state and national level. The Believe 271 Foundation Inc., a not for profit foundation, formed to help me with my fight, but now has turned to helping others, this team is here for you. Feel free to check us out at **www.believe271.com.** Our mission is to assist firefighters and their families who are battling cancer and life-threatening illnesses. In closing I must reiterate the fact that I would not be writing this book today, if it wasn't for my faith, family and friends. I will continue to fight the battle so that No One Will Ever Fight Alone Again.

CPSIA information can be obtained
at www.ICGtesting.com
Printed in the USA
BVOW07s0151271017
498807BV00010B/69/P